THE COMPLETE PLANT-BASED KITCHEN COOKBOOK FOR BEGINNERS

Nourishing Recipes for a Healthier You

Adam C.

DEDICATION

This book is dedicated to all my Readers

CONTENTS

Introduction

This is "The Complete Plant-Based Kitchen Cookbook for Beginners: Nourishing Recipes for a Healthier You." You will set out on a journey through the pages that come after to a healthier and kinder way of eating that honors the bounty of nature. With this cookbook, you may embark on a culinary journey where the wellbeing of your body and the environment coexist peacefully.

Concerning Plant-Based Eating

A lifestyle that emphasizes the consumption of complete, unprocessed foods made from plants is known as plant-based cooking. As a result, your plate's main ingredients will include vegetables, fruits, grains, legumes, nuts, seeds, and a variety of herbs and spices. Your meals will be tasty and nurturing thanks to the recipes in this book, which embrace the unique flavors, textures, and nutritional advantages that these ingredients offer.

The advantages of a plant-based diet

The benefits of switching to a plant-based diet are numerous and significant. It can enhance your general health as well as lower your carbon footprint and support animal welfare. By committing to a plant-based diet, you are moving significantly closer to:

- Reducing your risk of developing chronic conditions including diabetes, heart disease, and some types of cancer

- Getting to and keeping a healthy weight.

- Increasing your vitality and energy levels

- Maintaining our surroundings while doing so

- Supporting the treatment of animals humanely

Getting Started: Key Ingredients and Cooking Equipment

The idea of creating a plant-based pantry and obtaining the necessary kitchen equipment can be a bit intimidating for individuals who are new to plant-based cuisine. But do not worry; we will walk you through everything and give you the tools you need to begin the recipes. You'll learn about tools like high-speed blenders and vegetable spiralizers as well as necessary items like quinoa, nutritional yeast, and tahini that will make your transition to a plant-based diet both manageable and pleasurable.

Guides to Success

Any lifestyle change comes with its own set of difficulties, particularly when it involves food and nutrition. We have a section with success advice because of this. You may overcome potential challenges, such as dining out and food preparation, by using these useful suggestions. We'll offer advice to make sure your transition to a plant-based diet is not only scrumptious but also sustainable and fulfilling.

Remember that plant-based cuisine is not about deprivation as you begin this journey; rather, it's about embracing a world of flavors and options that will nourish your body and soul. Your guide on this journey is "The Complete Plant-Based Kitchen Cookbook for Beginners," a book full of nourishing dishes that will show how a plant-based diet can be both healthy and delectably tasty.

In order to achieve a better you, a healthier planet, and a world of culinary delights that await you on every page of this cookbook, let's begin this wonderful journey. Your health, your taste buds, and the environment as a whole will appreciate it.

Chapter 1: Breakfast treats

1.1 Overnight Creamy Oats

With our recipe for Creamy Overnight Oats, you can rise and shine to the delicious world of plant-based breakfasts. These oats are a divine combination of rolled oats, plant-based milk, and a variety of your favorite fruits, making them ideal for busy mornings. In addition to saving time, soaking them overnight yields a delicious, ready-to-eat breakfast that is rich in protein, fiber, and unrefined sugar.

Ingredients:

- Rolled oats, 1 cup
- 1 cup plant-based milk of your choosing, such as almond milk
- Two teaspoons of agave or maple syrup
- Vanilla extract, 1 teaspoon
- Sliced bananas, chopped almonds, and fresh berries as garnish

Instructions:

1. Combine the rolled oats, almond milk, maple syrup, and vanilla essence in a Mason jar or bowl.

2. Be sure to thoroughly stir the oats into the liquid.

3. Cover and chill for at least four hours or overnight.

4. Give it a good toss in the morning, then add chopped almonds, sliced bananas, and fresh berries for a delicious crunch.

1.2 Bowl of green smoothie

With our Green Smoothie Bowl, you can get your day off to a lively start. This dish not only tastes divine but is also a nutrient powerhouse thanks to its abundance of leafy greens, ripe fruits, and a boost of energy. You may use it as a blank canvas to express your creativity and top your smoothie bowl with anything you like, from granola and coconut flakes to fresh fruit and seeds.

Ingredients:

- Fresh spinach greens, 2 cups
- 1 frozen ripe banana

- 12 an avocado

- 1 cup plant-based milk of your choosing, such as almond milk

- Chia seeds, one tablespoon

- Toppings: Kiwi slices, oats, coconut shavings, and a honey or agave syrup drizzle

Instructions:

Blend spinach, frozen banana, avocado, almond milk, and chia seeds in a food processor.

Blend till creamy and smooth.

The smoothie should be poured into a bowl, and then topped as desired.

1.3 Veggie pancakes

Who says that eggs and dairy products are necessary to make fluffy, mouth-melting pancakes? Our vegan pancakes serve as evidence that the traditional breakfast dish may be enjoyed without using any animal products. These pancakes are the ideal weekend treat for you and your loved ones since they are fluffy, light, and wonderfully delicious.

Ingredients:

- All-purpose flour, 1 cup
- Two teaspoons of sugar
- 1 teaspoon of baking soda
- 1 cup almond milk (or any other plant-based milk of your choice) and 1/2 teaspoon salt
- Vegetable oil, two tablespoons
- Vanilla extract, 1 teaspoon

Instructions:

1. Mix the flour, sugar, baking soda, and salt in a sizable bowl.

2. The dry ingredients should be combined with the oil, vanilla extract, and almond milk. Don't over mix; just blend thoroughly.

3. A griddle or non-stick skillet heated to a medium-high temperature. For each pancake, pour 1/4 cup of batter.

4. Cook for two to three minutes, or until the pancake surface begins to bubble and the edges start to look set. Cook for a further two minutes, flipping once, or until golden brown.

5. Serve warm with maple syrup and your preferred plant-based butter.

1.4 Chia Seed Dessert

In this delicious Chia Seed Pudding recipe, the little nutritional powerhouses known as chia seeds take center stage. Chia seeds are turned into a creamy pudding that is not only filling but also high in omega-3 fatty acids, fiber, and antioxidants thanks to their capacity to absorb liquid and develop a gel-like consistency. Enjoy this pudding as a guilt-free dessert or for breakfast.

Ingredients:

- Chia seeds, 1/4 cup

- 1 cup plant-based milk of your choosing, such as almond milk

- 1 tablespoon of agave or maple syrup

- One-half teaspoon of vanilla extract

- Topping of fresh berries and sliced almonds

Instructions:

1. Chia seeds, almond milk, maple syrup, and vanilla essence should all be combined in a bowl.

2. To make sure the chia seeds are dispersed equally, whisk thoroughly.

3. Allow the mixture to thicken in the refrigerator for at least 2 hours or overnight.

4. Give it a thorough swirl just before serving. Add some delicious crunch by topping with sliced almonds and juicy berries.

1.5 Variations on avocado toast

The basic dish of avocado toast may be transformed in countless ways. By combining creamy avocado with a variety of delicious toppings, these variations on avocado toast will up your breakfast game while also adding flavor and texture.

Traditional avocado toast

On a slice of whole-grain toast, add mashed avocado, cherry tomatoes, red pepper flakes, and sea salt.

Toast with sweet and sour avocado:

On multigrain bread, there are mashed avocado, strawberry slices, balsamic sauce, and a sprinkle of honey.

Toasted Spicy Avocado:

On rye toast, there are mashed avocado, chopped radishes, cilantro, and a dash of red pepper flakes.

Avocado Toast Packed with Protein:

On whole-wheat toast, add mashed avocado, diced boiled eggs, black sesame seeds, and a dash of soy sauce.

Your mornings will be full with nourishment and excitement thanks to these delicious breakfast recipes. With a heart full of thanksgiving and a gut full of healthful plant-based delight, welcome the day. Enjoy your delicious breakfast, and get ready for the chapters that will feature even more nutritional meals!

Chapter 2: Delectable and Fresh Salads

Although they are frequently underrated, salads are anything but boring in the world of plant-based cooking. These colorful, nutrient-dense dishes demonstrate that a salad can stand alone as a filling, delectable, and substantial dinner. We'll look at a range of salads in this chapter that will not only tempt your taste senses but also leave you feeling filled and rejuvenated.

2.1 Traditional Garden Salad

Start with the traditional Classic Garden Salad. This salad, which is a straightforward yet delicious combination of fresh, crisp vegetables and greens, honors the beauty of nature's wealth. The secret is in the mixture of ingredients and the delicious dressing, which transforms the ordinary salad into a revitalizing work of art.

Ingredients:

To make the salad:

- Lettuce, spinach, arugula, and other mixed greens

- Cherry tomatoes, sliced Kalamata olives, julienned bell peppers, sliced cucumber, sliced red onion, and thinly sliced carrots

- Avocado, sunflower seeds or chickpeas are optional additions.

To be Dressed:

- Extra virgin olive oil, 3 teaspoons

- Balsamic vinegar, two tablespoons

- 1 minced garlic clove

- Dijon mustard, 1 teaspoon

- Pepper and salt as desired

Instructions:

1. Combine the mixed greens, cherry tomatoes, cucumber, red onion, carrots, bell peppers, and Kalamata olives in a sizable salad dish.

2. Mix the olive oil, balsamic vinegar, garlic powder, Dijon mustard, salt, and pepper to make the dressing.

3. Toss the salad with the dressing after drizzling it over it. Choose any optional add-ons you want to include.

4. Serve right away for a freshness boost.

2.2 Power Bowl of quinoa and chickpeas

The Quinoa and Chickpea Power Bowl is a healthy option for a salad that can be consumed as a meal in and of itself. This salad offers sustained energy and a pleasant medley of textures since it is loaded with protein-rich quinoa, fiber-rich chickpeas, and a variety of bright veggies.

Ingredients:

To make the salad:

- Cooked quinoa, 1 cup

- Fresh spinach or kale, cherry tomatoes, cucumber, sliced red onion, and 1 can of rinsed and drained chickpeas

- Sliced avocado

To be Dressed:

- Olive oil, 3 tablespoons

- Lemon juice, two tablespoons

- 1 teaspoon cumin powder 1 chopped garlic clove

- Pepper and salt as desired

Instructions:

1. The cooked quinoa, chickpeas, cucumber, red onion, cherry tomatoes, and fresh greens should all be combined in a big bowl.

2. Slices of avocado may be added.

3. Mix the olive oil, lemon juice, ground cumin, minced garlic, salt, and pepper to make the dressing.

4. Over the salad, drizzle the dressing, and mix to blend.

5. Enjoy this nutritious lunch.

2.3 Colorful Detox Salad

The colorful and flavorful Rainbow Detox Salad detoxifies your body while titillating your taste buds. This colorful concoction of vegetables and herbs is a great way to refresh and rejuvenate your body.

Ingredients:

To make the salad:

- Shredded carrots and finely sliced red cabbage

- Thinly sliced green beans, blanched red and yellow bell peppers, and thinly sliced red bell pepper

- Chopped fresh cilantro

- Brand-new mint leaves

To be Dressed:

- Rice vinegar, two tablespoons

- 1 tablespoon of Tamari or soy sauce

- Sesame oil, 1 teaspoon

- 1 teaspoon of maple syrup or honey

- 1/8 teaspoon grated fresh ginger

Instructions:

1. Red cabbage, grated carrots, red and yellow bell peppers, blanched green beans, cilantro, and mint leaves should all be combined in a big bowl.

2. Mix the rice vinegar, soy sauce, sesame oil, honey or maple syrup, and shredded ginger in a bowl to make the dressing.

3. Toss the salad with the dressing after drizzling it over it. Prior to serving, give the salad some time to marinate.

2.4 Salad in the Mediterranean with tofu feta

This delicious salad will take your taste senses to the Mediterranean coast. Fresh veggies and marinated tofu are combined in the Mediterranean Salad with Tofu Feta for a taste explosion. It is the ideal illustration of how conventional flavors may be replicated using plant-based ingredients.

Ingredients:

To make the salad:

- Chopped Romaine lettuce, cherry tomatoes, cucumbers, red onions, and thinly sliced Kalamata olives

- Tofu feta (Includes recipe)

Regarding the tofu feta:

- 1 box cubed, drained extra-firm tofu

- Olive oil, two tablespoons

- Lemon juice, two tablespoons

- 1 minced garlic clove

- Oregano, dry, 1 teaspoon

- Pepper and salt as desired

Instructions:

1. Cubed tofu, olive oil, lemon juice, minced garlic, dried oregano, salt, and pepper are all ingredients in the tofu feta. Allow to marinate for at least 30 minutes while gently tossing to coat.

2. Chop the romaine lettuce and blend it with the cherry tomatoes, cucumber, red onion, and Kalamata olives in a big salad bowl.

3. Top the salad with the marinated tofu feta.

4. Over the salad, drizzle the tofu-feta marinade.

5. Serve this delicious Mediterranean dish after a gentle toss.

2.5 Cashew-dressed Caesar salad

A traditional Caesar salad without anchovies, dairy, or eggs with our Caesar Salad with Cashew Dressing, it is indeed feasible. This salad's famed creamy cashew-based dressing, which has the ideal mingling of tastes, is a game-changer.

Ingredients:

To make the salad:

- Romaine lettuce, homemade or store-bought chopped croutons, and whole-grain bread

- (Homemade or store-bought) Vegan Parmesan cheese

- When making the cashew Caesar dressing:

- 1 cup raw cashews, drained after soaking for two to four hours

- 7/8 cup of water

- Lemon juice, two tablespoons

- One garlic clove

- 1/9 cup nutritional yeast

- Dijon mustard, 1 teaspoon

- Pepper and salt as desired

Instructions:

3 Blend the soaked cashews, water, lemon juice, garlic, nutritional yeast, Dijon mustard, salt, and pepper to produce the Cashew Caesar Dressing. If necessary, add more water to change the consistency.

4 Combine the romaine lettuce, croutons, and Vegan Parmesan cheese in a big bowl.

5 Over the salad, drizzle the Cashew Caesar Dressing and toss to combine.

6 Enjoy the creamy, dairy-free richness of this Caesar salad when you serve it with a twist.

These salads show off the variety, flavors, and inventiveness of plant-based cooking and are more than just appetizers. These dishes, which range from the classic Garden Salad to the creative Caesar Salad with Cashew Dressing, demonstrate that salads can be incredibly delicious and nutritious. Investigate these choices and welcome the vitality and health they add to your menu.

Chapter 3: Hearty Soups and Stews

Soups and stews are the best comfort foods, in my opinion. We go into the world of comforting soups and stews made from plants in this chapter, which will not only warm your belly but also your soul. These dishes offer a symphony of tastes and textures, from time-honored classics to works of art that draw inspiration from around the world.

3.1 Spaghetti Squash

Known for being filling and healthy, minestrone is a popular Italian soup. It's a harmonious medley of perfectly cooked vegetables, beans, and pasta. In addition to being cholesterol-free, our plant-based minestrone soup recipe has all the flavor and heartiness of the classic recipe.

Ingredients:

- One tablespoon of olive oil

- 1 onion, diced; 2 carrots, diced; 4 celery stalks, minced; 1 zucchini, diced; and 1 can of kidney beans, drained and washed

- Diced tomatoes in one can

- One cup of chopped green beans in six cups of vegetable broth

- Elbow macaroni or ditalini, one cup of tiny pasta

- A tsp. of dried oregano

- As desired, add salt and pepper.

- A garnish of fresh basil leaves

- As a garnish and optional, vegan Parmesan cheese

Instructions:

2   Over medium heat, warm the olive oil in a big pot. Include the onion, celery, carrots, and garlic. About 5 minutes of sautéing should soften the vegetables.

3   Vegetable broth, dried oregano, green beans, kidney beans, and chopped tomatoes should all be added. Bring to a boil before turning down the heat and allowing it to simmer for 15 to 20 minutes.

4   As directed on the package, add the pasta and cook it until al

dente.

5   To taste, add salt and pepper to the soup.

6   Serve hot with optional Vegan Parmesan cheese and fresh

basil leaves as garnish.

3.2 Stew with Lentils and Veggies

Our lentil and vegetable stew's major ingredient, lentils are an
excellent source of fiber and plant-based protein. Rich, filling,
and nutritious goodness abound in this stew. When you need
something to warm you from the inside out on a cool evening,
this recipe is ideal.

Ingredients:

- One tablespoon of olive oil

- Diced one onion

- 2 diced carrots, 2 diced celery stalks, and 2 minced cloves
  of garlic

- Brown or green lentils, 1 cup

- Tomato dice from one can

- Two bay leaves, six cups of vegetable broth

- 1 tsp. dried thyme

- To taste with salt and pepper

- Garnishing with fresh parsley

Instructions:

2 Over medium heat, warm the olive oil in a big pot. Include the onion, celery, carrots, and garlic. About 5 minutes of sautéing should soften the vegetables.

3 Add the bay leaves, dried thyme, salt, pepper, lentils, diced tomatoes, and vegetable broth.

4 The mixture should be heated to a rolling boil before being simmered for 30 to 40 minutes, depending on how tender you like your lentils.

5 Take out and throw away the bay leaves.

6 Garnish with fresh parsley before serving hot.

3.3 Coconut Curry Soup in Thailand

With our Thai Coconut Curry Soup, you can transport your taste buds to the vivacious streets of Thailand. The coconut milk, red curry paste, and a variety of fresh vegetables are harmoniously combined in this flavorful and aromatic soup. You won't want to miss this adventure through flavors and spices.

Ingredients:

- Red curry paste, 1 tablespoon

- One can of coconut milk

- 1 julienned carrot in 3 cups of vegetable broth

- One thinly sliced red bell pepper and one thinly sliced or spiralized zucchini

- 100 grams of broccoli florets

- One cup of snap peas

- Sliced mushrooms in a cup and diced extra-firm tofu in a block

- One lime juice

- Lime wedges and fresh cilantro, for garnish

Instructions:

2   For one to two minutes, cook the red curry paste in a big pot on medium heat.

3   Vegetable broth and coconut milk should be added. Mix everything thoroughly.

4   You should also include the tofu, carrot, red bell pepper, zucchini, broccoli, and snap peas. The vegetables should be soft after 15 to 20 minutes of simmering.

5   Add lime juice and stir.

6   Serve hot, topped with lime wedges and chopped cilantro.

3.4 Chili Black Beans with Heat

Our Spicy Black Bean Chili is no exception to the rule that chili is the definition of comfort food. This chili will fill you up while pleasing your palate because it is loaded with protein, fiber, and strong tastes. This recipe is ideal for gatherings or winter nights at home.

Ingredients:

- 1 teaspoon of olive oil

- Diced one onion

- Minced garlic from 2 cloves

- Chopped red bell pepper, one

- A single chopped green bell pepper

- One minced jalapeno pepper, to taste

- Drained and washed black beans from one can

- Drained and washed kidney beans from one can

- Tomato dice from one can

- Fresh or frozen corn kernels, 1 cup

- Two tablespoons of chili powder per three cups of vegetable broth

- 1 tsp. of cumin

- To taste with salt and pepper

- For garnish (optional), add fresh cilantro and vegan sour cream.

Instructions:

2 Over medium heat, warm the olive oil in a big pot. Add the red, green, and jalapeo peppers, as well as the onion and garlic. About 5 minutes of sautéing should soften the vegetables.

3   Add the vegetable broth, diced tomatoes, corn, black beans, kidney beans, cumin, chili powder, and salt and pepper.

4   The mixture is heated until it boils, then the heat is turned down, and it simmers for 30 to 40 minutes.

5   If desired, top with a dollop of vegan sour cream and fresh cilantro before serving.

3.5 Delicious Potato-Leek Soup

Classic Creamy Potato Leek Soup has been given a plant-based makeover. This creamy, fatty soup is pleasant and calming. It embodies comfort food at its finest and demonstrates that you don't need dairy to make opulently creamy soup.

Ingredients:

- 2 teaspoons of olive oil
- 2 leeks cleaned and sliced into the white and light green halves.
- 3 big potatoes, chopped and peeled
- Four cups of vegetable stock
- 0.5 teaspoons of dried thyme and 1 bay leaf

- To taste with salt and pepper

- To garnish: fresh chives

- Optional topping: vegan sour cream

Instructions:

2 Over medium heat, warm the olive oil in a big pot. Sliced leeks should be added and sautéed for about 5 minutes, or until tender and transparent.

3 Add the vegetable broth, bay leaf, dried thyme, salt, and pepper along with the cubed potatoes.

4 When the potatoes are cooked, simmer the mixture for 20 to 25 minutes after bringing it to a boil.

5 Take out and throw away the bay leaf.

6 To make the soup smooth and creamy, purée it using an immersion blender, alternately, add the soup in portions and puree the mixture until smooth.

7 If desired, top with a dollop of vegan sour cream and fresh chives before serving.

Every spoonful of these warming soups and stews will comfort and warm you. They are the ideal addition to your plant-based kitchen. You can choose from a variety of dishes to suit your taste and mood, ranging from the Italian-inspired Minestrone to the hot kick of the hot Black Bean Chili. These dishes not only nourish us but also bring back the delight of a satisfying bowl of soup.

Chapter 4: Delicious Main Courses

This chapter explores a wide range of filling and robust plant-based main courses that highlight the variety of tastes and textures found in plant-based cooking. These dishes demonstrate how flexible and delicious plant-based cooking can be, ranging from international classics to avant-garde inventions.

4.1 Chickpea curry with masala

With the help of our Chickpea Tikka Masala, you can bring a taste of India into your home. This recipe mixes delicate chickpeas with a flavorful tomato-based sauce that has been flavored with a variety of savory spices. It's a hit with the crowd and will keep you going back for more.

Ingredients:

- Cooked chickpeas, two cups
- 1 finely chopped onion
- 2 minced garlic cloves
- Minced ginger, 1 inch long

- 1 tomato diced can

- Full-fat coconut milk in one can.

- Tomato paste, two tablespoons

- Garam masala, 1 1/2 tablespoons

- 1 teaspoon each of ground cumin and coriander

- One-half teaspoon of ground turmeric

- 0.5 teaspoons of chili powder, tasted,

- Pepper and salt as desired

- For garnish: fresh cilantro

- Naan bread or cooked rice for serving

Instructions:

2 The chopped onion, garlic, and ginger should be sautéed in a big pan until they are fragrant and transparent.

3 Add the tomato paste, coconut milk, diced tomatoes, and all the seasonings. To blend, thoroughly stir.

4 Once the sauce has thickened and the cooked chickpeas are well heated, add the chickpeas that have already been cooked.

5 To taste, add salt and pepper to the food.

6   Serve hot with fresh cilantro over top of cooked rice or with

naan bread.

4.2 Steaks with portobello mushrooms

The delicious vegan substitute for conventional steak is these portobello mushroom steaks. They provide a meaty texture and a savory umami flavor when marinated in a delicious combination and cooked to perfection. They are ideal for a casual dinner at home or a plant-based BBQ.

Ingredients:

- Removed stems from 4 big Portobello mushrooms

- Balsamic vinegar, 1/4 cup

- 2 tablespoons of Tamari or soy sauce

- 2 minced garlic cloves

- One tablespoon of dried thyme

- Pepper and salt as desired

- Grilling with olive oil

Instructions:

2   Balsamic vinegar, soy sauce, minced garlic, dried thyme, salt, and pepper should all be combined in a bowl.

3   Pour the marinade over the Portobello mushrooms after placing them in a shallow dish. Allow them to marinade for at least 30 minutes while occasionally stirring them.

4   Lightly oil a grill or grill pan and preheat it over medium-high heat.

5   The marinated Portobello mushrooms should be grilled for 5 to 7 minutes on each side, or until they are soft and have grill marks.

6   Serve warm alongside your preferred side dishes.

4.3 Pasta with a lentil bolognese sauce

A traditional Italian staple with a plant-based twist is our spaghetti with lentil bolognese. Pasta and the hearty lentil sauce provide a filling dinner that is high in protein and flavor. It's the ideal option for a homey evening in or a family dinner.

Ingredients:

- Cooked brown or green lentils, 2 cups

- 1 finely chopped onion

- 2 minced garlic cloves

- 1 carrot, cut finely

- 1 celery stalk, cut finely

- 1 tomato diced can

- Tomato paste, two tablespoons

- Oregano, dry, 1 teaspoon

- A half-teaspoon of dried basil

- Pepper and salt as desired

- Vegan Parmesan cheese for topping (Optional)

- Garnished with fresh basil

Instructions:

1. To blend, thoroughly stir.

4.3 Sweet Potato and Black Bean Enchiladas

Enchiladas are a Mexican comfort food that's taken to the next level with our Sweet Potato and Black Bean Enchiladas. These enchiladas feature a filling of sweet potatoes and black beans, wrapped in corn tortillas and smothered in a rich and spicy enchilada sauce. They are a delightful blend of sweet and savory, creating a meal that's both satisfying and nutritious.

Ingredients:

- 2 large sweet potatoes, peeled and diced
- 1 can black beans, drained and rinsed
- 1 teaspoon ground cumin
- 1/2 teaspoon chili powder
- Salt and pepper to taste
- 12 corn tortillas
- 2 cups enchilada sauce
- 1 cup vegan cheese, shredded (optional)
- Fresh cilantro, for garnish

Instructions:

2. Preheat your oven to 375°F (190°C).

3. In a large bowl, combine the diced sweet potatoes, black beans, ground cumin, chili powder, salt, and pepper.

4. Steam or boil the sweet potatoes until they are tender, then mash them into the bean mixture.

5. Warm the corn tortillas for a few seconds in a dry skillet or microwave.

6. Place a spoonful of the sweet potato and black bean mixture in each tortilla, roll them up, and place them seam-side down in a baking dish.

7. Pour the enchilada sauce over the rolled tortillas, and sprinkle with vegan cheese, if desired.

8. Bake for about 20-25 minutes, or until the enchiladas are heated through and the cheese is melted (if using)

9. Garnish with fresh cilantro before serving.

These wholesome main dishes showcase the incredible variety of plant-based options for satisfying and delicious meals. From the rich flavors of Chickpea Tikka Masala to the hearty simplicity of Portobello Mushroom Steaks, you'll find a wide range of dishes to explore and enjoy. Embrace the world of plant-based cuisine and discover the creativity it offers for nourishing main courses.

Chapter 5: Filling Sides and Snacks

Any meal's unsung heroes are its sides and snacks. We look at a variety of delicious and filling plant-based options in this chapter. These dishes are ideal for sharing with friends, serving as a side dish with your main course, or simply enjoying on their own.

5.1 Fried Sweet Potatoes in the Oven

Baked sweet potato fries, a deliciously sweet and savory alternative to regular fries, are now available. These fries are not only delicious, but also a better choice for your health than regular fries. They are excellent on their own as a snack or as a side dish.

Ingredients:

- Fries made from two large sweet potatoes that have been peeled

- 2 teaspoons of olive oil

- Paprika, 1 teaspoon

- 50% of a teaspoon of garlic powder

- To taste with salt and pepper

- Garnishing with fresh parsley

Instructions:

1. Put a baking sheet in the oven and preheat it to 425 °F (220 °C).

2. Sweet potato fries should be well-coated in a large bowl with olive oil, paprika, garlic powder, salt, and pepper.

3. On the preheated baking sheet, spread the fries in a single layer.

4. Fries should be baked until crispy and golden, about 25 to 30 minutes, flipping them halfway through.

5. Garnish with fresh parsley before serving hot.

5.2 Avocado and salsa

Guacamole and salsa are a must-have for any gathering because they make a classic pairing. Salsa's zesty freshness and the creamy richness of guacamole go together beautifully. These are excellent sauces to serve with tacos, tortilla chips, or as a side dish with many Mexican-inspired dishes.

Ingredients for guacamole:

- 2 mature avocados, peeled and pitted
- 1 clove of minced garlic, 1/4 cup finely chopped red onion, 1 tomato, diced
- 1 lime's worth of juice 1/4 cup chopped cilantro
- To taste with salt and pepper

Salsa Ingredients:

- 3 diced tomatoes, 1 minced jalapeno (adjust to taste), 1/2 finely chopped onion, and 1/4 cup chopped cilantro.
- One lime juice
- To taste with salt and pepper

Instructions:

1. Avocados should be mashed before being combined with red onion, minced garlic, diced tomato, cilantro, lime juice, salt, and pepper to make guacamole. Make a good mixture.

2. Combine the minced jalapenos, cilantro, finely chopped onion, diced tomatoes, lime juice, salt, and pepper to make the salsa. Mix thoroughly by stirring.

3. Serve the salsa and guacamole in separate bowls, or layer them together to make a vibrant and flavorful dip.

5.3 Dip made without animal products

One dish that is sure to please everyone is vegan spinach artichoke dip. This dip is flavorful and creamy, making it ideal for dipping tortilla chips, raw vegetables, or spreading on your preferred bread or crackers

Ingredients:

- 1 (10-ounce) package of thawed and drained frozen chopped spinach

- Artichoke hearts from one (14-ounce) can, drained and chopped

- One-half cup vegan cream cheese

- A half-cup of vegan mayonnaise

- A half-cup of vegan Parmesan cheese

- One-fourth cup nutritional yeast

- Minced garlic from 2 cloves

- To taste with salt and pepper

Instructions:

1. 350°F (175°C) should be the oven's temperature.

2. Spinach that has been drained, chopped artichoke hearts, vegan cream cheese, vegan mayonnaise, vegan Parmesan cheese, nutritional yeast, minced garlic, salt, and pepper should all be combined in a big bowl, make a good mixture.

3. Bake the mixture in a baking dish for 25 to 30 minutes, or until it is hot and bubbling.

4. Serve warm with your preferred dippers.

5.4 Crispy Bites of Buffalo Cauliflower

Crispy Buffalo Cauliflower Bites are an enticing and spicily delicious snack that is ideal for game day or whenever you're in the mood for something spicy. Instead of traditional Buffalo wings, try these tasty and healthier cauliflower bites.

Ingredients:

- Cut one head of cauliflower into bite-sized florets.

- All-purpose flour, 1 cup (or chickpea flour for a gluten-free option)

- Water, 1 cup

- Garlic powder, 1 teaspoon

- One tablespoon of onion powder

- To taste with salt and pepper

- 1/2 cup hot sauce, taste-tested

- Two tablespoons of vegan butter, along with optional vegan ranch or blue cheese dressing, for dipping

Instructions:

1. Set a baking sheet on the bottom of the oven and preheat it to 450°F (230°C).

2. Make a batter by combining the flour, water, garlic powder, onion powder, salt, and pepper in a large bowl.

3. Place each cauliflower floret on the lined baking sheet after dipping it into the batter and letting any excess drip off.

4. The cauliflower should be baked for 20 to 25 minutes, or until it is crisp and golden.

5. Melted vegan butter and hot sauce should be combined in a different bowl. Sprinkle this mixture evenly over the baked cauliflower.

6. Serve hot, if desired with vegan ranch or blue cheese dressing for dipping.

5.5 Brussels sprouts roasted with garlic

An easy but flavorful side dish for any occasion is garlic-roasted Brussels sprouts. Roasted Brussels sprouts and garlic combine to make a delicious dish that is also filling and healthy.

Ingredients:

- 1 pound of halved and trimmed Brussels sprouts

- 4 minced garlic cloves

- 2 teaspoons of olive oil

- To taste with salt and pepper

- Lemon zest as a garnish, if desired

Instructions:

1. Put a baking sheet in the oven and preheat it to 400 °F (200 °C).

2. Combine the chopped garlic, olive oil, salt, and pepper in a bowl with the halved Brussels sprouts.

3. On the baking sheet that has been prepared, spread the Brussels sprouts in a single layer.

4. Roast for 20 to 25 minutes or until the edges are crispy and the vegetables are tender.

5. Before serving, if desired, garnish with lemon zest.

You can enhance the flavor and variety of your plant-based meals with these filling sides and snacks. You can choose from dishes to broaden your culinary horizons, such as the irresistible Baked Sweet Potato Fries and the zingy Guacamole and Salsa. Discover the joy of wholesome and mouthwatering sides by embracing the world of plant-based snacking.

Chapter 6: Delectable Desserts

Without a satisfying dessert, no meal is complete, and plant-based cuisine is no different. We'll look at a variety of delicious desserts in this chapter that are both indulgent and nourishing. These dessert recipes will allow you to maintain your plant-based diet while also satisfying your sweet tooth.

6.1 Vegan Avocado Chocolate Mousse

Enjoy the rich, creamy flavor of the vegan chocolate avocado mousse. This dessert combines the natural goodness of avocados with the decadence of chocolate for a decadent and guilt-free treat. It's ideal for those who enjoy chocolate and want a healthier dessert option.

Ingredients:

- Peeled and pitted two ripe avocados.

- Unsweetened cocoa powder, 1/4 cup

- 1/4 cup agave nectar or maple syrup

- Vanilla extract, 1 teaspoon

- A dash of salt

- As a garnish, you can use shaved chocolate or fresh berries.

Instructions:

1. The ripe avocados, unsweetened cocoa powder, maple syrup or agave nectar, vanilla extract, and a dash of salt should all be combined in a blender or food processor.

2. Blend the mixture until it's creamy and smooth.

3. Place portions of the mousse in serving bowls.

4. Before serving, let the food cool for at least 30 minutes in the refrigerator.

5. If desired, garnish with sliced chocolate or fresh berries.

6.2 A fruit crisp with oats on top

A delightful and soothing dessert that honors the inherent sweetness of fresh berries is berry crisp with oat topping. This crisp has a juicy berry filling and a crunchy oat-based topping. It's the ideal way to take pleasure in the seasonal flavors.

Ingredients:

The Filling:

- 4 cups of mixed berries, including raspberries, blueberries, and strawberries

- 1/4 cup agave nectar or maple syrup

- 1 tablespoon arrowroot powder or corn starch

- 1/8 cup lemon juice

Regarding the Topping

- Rolled oats, 1 cup

- For a gluten-free option, use oat flour in place of half a cup of whole wheat flour.

- One-fourth cup coconut sugar

- A quarter cup of melted coconut oil

- Half a teaspoon of cinnamon

- A dash of salt

Instructions:

1. Turn on the oven to 350 °F (175 °C).

2. The mixed berries, maple syrup or agave nectar, corn starch or arrowroot powder, and lemon juice should all be combined in a bowl. Add to a baking dish after thoroughly mixing.

3. Rolling oats, whole wheat flour, coconut sugar, melted coconut oil, cinnamon, and a dash of salt should all be combined in a different bowl until crumbly, combine.

4. The berry mixture in the baking dish should be covered with the oat topping.

5. Bake for about 25 to 30 minutes, or until the berries are bubbling and the topping is golden.

6. Serve warm with a dollop of coconut whipped cream or a scoop of vegan ice cream.

6.3 Walnut and Banana Muffins

A traditional favorite with a plant-based twist are banana walnut muffins. These muffins are full of the goodness of ripe bananas and crunchy walnuts, and they are moist and flavorful. They make a delicious snack or breakfast food.

Ingredients:

- 2 mashed ripe bananas

- 1/4 cup agave nectar or maple syrup

- 14 cup of plain applesauce

- 1/4 cup of plant-based milk, such as almond milk

- Vanilla extract, 1 teaspoon

- A gluten-free alternative to whole wheat flour is oat flour.

- One tablespoon of baking soda

- Half a teaspoon of cinnamon

- 14 teaspoon of salt

- Chopped walnuts, half a cup

Instructions:

1. Paper liners should be used to line a muffin tin as your oven is preheated to 350°F (175°C).

2. The mashed bananas, maple syrup or agave nectar, unsweetened applesauce, almond milk, and vanilla extract should all be combined in a bowl. Mix thoroughly.

3. Mix the whole wheat flour, baking soda, cinnamon, and salt in a different bowl.

4. Just combine the dry ingredients with the addition of the wet ingredients.

5. Add the chopped walnuts slowly and gently.

6. Fill each muffin cup about two-thirds full after dividing the batter among them.

7. When a toothpick is inserted into the center of a muffin, it should come out clean after 20 to 25 minutes of baking.

8. Before serving, allow the muffins to cool.

6.4 Date and Coconut Energy Balls

The ideal dessert or snack for when you need a quick boost of energy is a coconut date energy ball. Dates, nuts, and coconut are used to make these healthy no-bake treats. They make delicious on-the-go snacks because they are sweet and filling.

Ingredients:

- 1 cup dates with pits
- Oats, rolled, in a cup

- 1/2 cup coconut shavings

- 1/2 cup cashews or almonds

- Cocoa powder, 1/4 cup

- Quarter cup of almond butter

- Vanilla extract, 1 teaspoon

- A dash of salt

Instructions:

1. In a food processor, combine all the ingredients and process until the mixture comes together and becomes sticky.

2. Roll the mixture's small balls between your hands as you shape them.

3. Refrigerate the energy balls for about 30 minutes to set them, then place them on a tray lined with parchment paper.

4. Transfer them to an airtight container and place them in the refrigerator once they are firm.

6.5 Vegetarian Cheesecake

A dairy-free dessert that is creamy and dreamy is plant-based cheesecake. This recipe offers a vegan twist on the traditional cheesecake and makes a rich, decadent treat that's ideal for celebrations or just when you're craving something special.

Ingredients:

Within the Crust:

- 1 and a half cups almond flour

- Melted 1/4 cup coconut oil and 2 tablespoons of agave nectar or maple syrup

The Filling:

- 2 cups of uncooked cashews soaked for two hours in hot water

- 50 ml of coconut cream

- 50 ml of lemon juice

- 1/2 cup agave nectar or maple syrup

- A quarter cup of melted coconut oil

- Vanilla extract, 1 teaspoon

- A dash of salt

- For garnish, use fresh berries.

Instructions:

1. For best results, line a spring form pan with parchment paper and preheat the oven to 350°F (175°C).

2. Almond flour, melted coconut oil, and maple syrup or agave nectar should all be combined in a bowl. The crust is made by pressing this mixture into the bottom of the pan that has been prepared.

3. The soaked cashews, coconut cream, lemon juice, maple syrup or agave nectar, melted coconut oil, vanilla extract, and a dash of salt should all be combined in a blender. Blend the mixture until it's creamy and smooth.

4. Spread the filling evenly over the crust after pouring it on.

5. Bake for 45 to 50 minutes or until the center is just barely jiggly and the edges are golden.

6. Refrigerate the cheesecake for at least 4 hours or overnight to set, and then allow it to cool to room temperature.

7. If desired, garnish with fresh berries before serving.

Your plant-based meals can be sweetly concluded32++ with one of these delectable sweets. You'll find options that satiate your sweet tooth while maintaining a plant-based and healthful diet, from the decadence of Vegan Chocolate Avocado Mousse to the fruity delight of Berry Crisp. Enjoy these guilt-free plant-based treats!

Chapter 7: Beverages and Smoothies

You must drink hydrating, nourishing beverages to go with your plant-based meals. This chapter introduces a variety of energizing beverages and smoothies that will keep you hydrated, revitalized, and energized all day long. You can choose from a variety of options to suit your preferences and needs, ranging from cleansing green smoothies to energizing morning elixirs.

7.1 Green Smoothie for Detox

Start your day off right with a green detox smoothie that is loaded with fruit and vegetables that are high in nutrients. This energizing mixture not only tastes great but also aids in body detoxification and renewal. It's a great way to increase your energy while receiving a balanced serving of vitamins and antioxidants.

Ingredients:

- One cup of new spinach

- Half a cucumber

- 1 cored and chopped green apple

- Juiced lemon, half

- 1/2 cup coconut water or water

- 1 teaspoon of optional chia seeds

- Ice cubes to make it even colder (optional)

Instructions:

1. In a blender, combine the fresh spinach, cucumber, green apple, lemon juice, and water.

2. Blend the ingredients together thoroughly and smoothly.

3. Add chia seeds and blend the smoothie once more for a thicker consistency.

4. Add some ice cubes and blend once more for added chill.

5. In a glass, pour the green detox smoothie and savor its energizing flavor.

7.2 Nutella Milk

Almond milk is a flexible plant-based milk substitute that is excellent for use in smoothies, recipes, and drinking on its own. It naturally lacks dairy and is a fantastic source of calcium.

Ingredients:

- 1 cup of overnight soaked raw almonds

- Water in 4 cups

- Choice of sweetener (optional): dates, agave nectar, or maple syrup

- 1 teaspoon optional vanilla extract

Instructions:

1. The almonds should be drained and rinsed.

2. Blend the almonds that have been soaked in water.

3. For two to three minutes, blend until smooth

4. Pour the mixture into a clean container after straining it through a nut milk bag, fine cheesecloth, or a fine-mesh strainer.

5. If desired, add vanilla extract after sweetening with your preferred sweetener.

6. For up to 4-5 days, keep your homemade almond milk in the fridge.

7.3 Herbal iced teas

Stay energized with a selection of delicious, caffeine-free iced herbal teas. Herbal teas come in a wide variety of flavors and advantages, making them a great option for a soothing afternoon or as a cool substitute for sweet drinks.

Ingredients:

- Herbal tea bags of your choice, such as peppermint, chamomile, hibiscus, and lavender

- Warm water

- An ice cube

- Sweetener (optional): stevia, honey, or agave nectar

- Slices of fresh fruit or lemon are optional.

Instructions:

1. Prepare your preferred herbal tea by steeping tea bags in hot water as directed on the package.

2. Wait until the tea is at room temperature.

3. After it has cooled, put the tea in the fridge to chill for a few hours.

4. Pour the chilled herbal tea over the ice in a glass, garnish with fruit slices if desired, and serve immediately.

5. Iced herbal tea that has been naturally sweetened after stirring

7.4 Elixir for an Energizing Morning

An energizing morning elixir that combines the advantages of warm water, lemon, and a hint of natural sweetness can help you get your day started. This potion can jump-start your metabolism and give you a boost of energy without the use of coffee.

Ingredients:

- 1-cup of hot water

- Lemon juice from a half

- 1 teaspoon agave nectar or maple syrup

- 1/8 teaspoon cinnamon powder

- A pinch of cayenne pepper for added heat (Optional)

1. Warm water, lemon juice, maple syrup or agave nectar, ground cinnamon, and cayenne pepper, if you like it hot, should all be combined in a mug.

2. Till everything dissolves, thoroughly stir.

3. For a healthy start to the day and to wake up your digestive system, sip your energizing morning elixir before breakfast.

7.5 Strawberry Smoothie

The Berry Blast Smoothie is an energizing and antioxidant-rich concoction of mixed berries that is ideal for a quick breakfast or a pick-me-up in the middle of the day. This smoothie has a delicious flavor from the combination of sweet and tart flavors.

Ingredients:

- Strawberries, blueberries, and raspberries in a cup of mixed frozen berries

- One ripe banana

- 1 cup plant-based milk, such as oat, almond, or soy milk

- Chia seeds, one tablespoon

- 1 teaspoon maple syrup or agave nectar (optional)

Instructions:

1. Blend together the mixed frozen berries, banana that has reached peak ripeness, plant-based milk, chia seeds, and sweetener of choice.

2. Blend the mixture until it's creamy and smooth.

3. Enjoy the delicious and vibrant flavors by pouring the Berry Blast Smoothie into a glass.

These drinks and smoothies provide a delicious range of options that will keep you hydrated and energized all day. You'll find a variety of hydrating and nourishing drinks that fit your plant-based lifestyle, from the detoxifying qualities of the Green Detox Smoothie to the calming effect of Iced Herbal Teas. Salutations to good health!

Chapter 8: Lifestyle Advice and Meal Planning

Changing to a plant-based diet requires more than just recipe knowledge. The strategies for meal preparation and lifestyle advice in this chapter will help you succeed in your transition to a plant-based diet.

8.1 Weekly Meal Schedule

An essential component of successful plant-based eating is making a weekly meal plan. You can maintain organization, ensure a healthy diet, and cut down on food waste. Here is a quick method for making your weekly meal plan:

1. Examine Your Schedule: Consider your work, school, and family commitments as you review the upcoming week. Determine the days you have more time to prepare meals and the days you need quick and simple fare.

2. Decide on Your Meals: Choose a few meals for the following week for breakfast, lunch, and dinner. To keep things interesting, use a variety of ingredients and cuisines.

3. Prepare extra portions to have leftovers for later meals, cutting down on cooking time and preventing food waste.

4. Think about Convenience: For hectic days, keep quick-to-prepare options on hand, such as overnight oats for breakfast or pre-chopped vegetables for salads.

5. Write It Down: List your planned meals for the coming week in a journal or using a meal planning app.

6. Make a shopping list based on your meal plan and the ingredients you will require. To avoid making impulsive purchases, stick to the list.

8.2 Plant-based ingredient shopping

To make the process simpler and more effective, remember these suggestions when looking for plant-based ingredients:

- Explore the produce section and add a variety of fresh fruits and vegetables to your shopping cart. For optimum affordability and freshness, choose seasonal produce.

- Choose Whole Grains: To get the necessary fiber and nutrients, choose whole grains like brown rice, quinoa, whole wheat pasta, and oats.

- Stock up on plant-based protein sources like beans, lentils, tofu, tempeh, and nuts for maximum protein power.

- Alternatives to dairy products include plant-based milks like almond, soy, or oat milk as well as dairy-free cheese and yogurt.

- When buying packaged foods, carefully read the labels to look for ingredients derived from animals.

- Spices and herbs: To flavor your food without using too much salt or unhealthy seasonings, invest in a variety of spices and herbs.

- Maintain a supply of frozen fruits and vegetables for smoothies and quick meal additions.

- Don't forget to stock up on water and herbal teas to stay hydrated.

8.3 Going Out and Eating Plant-Based

With a few tips, eating out as a plant-based eater can be fun and stress-free:

- Plan Ahead: Before you go, check the menu online to see if there are any plant-based options.

- Customize Your Order: If you want to make an item on the menu plant-based, don't be afraid to request substitutions or omissions.

- Ask Questions: If you have any questions about the ingredients, don't be afraid to ask your server or the chef.

- Ethnic Cuisine: Try eating at establishments that specialize in international cuisines like Indian, Thai, or Mediterranean, which frequently have a wide variety of plant-based dishes.

- Fast food: Even fast food franchises now provide vegetarian and vegan options like veggie burgers. When you're on the go, these can be an easy option.

8.4 Overcoming Typical Obstacles

You may face some difficulties as you travel your plant-based journey. This is how to get past them:

- In social situations, let your friends and family know about your dietary preferences and recommend plant-based eateries or potluck dishes.

- Cravings: Try substituting some of your favorite non-vegan foods with ones made of plants, and keep in mind that cravings for animal products usually lessen over time.

- Nutritional Concerns: Eat a variety of plant-based foods to make sure you're getting all the nutrients you need. Consider taking a B12 supplement, and if necessary, seek advice from a registered dietitian.

- Time constraints: Use batch cooking to prepare meals ahead of time and plan quick and simple meals for busy days.

- Food Labels: Read food labels carefully and become familiar with common animal ingredients that are hidden on them, such as rennet, casein, and gelatin.

8.5 Sustainable Development and Moral Issues

Eating a plant-based diet has a positive impact on the environment and animal welfare in addition to one's own health:

- Environmental Impact: Compared to an animal-based diet, a plant-based diet is more environmentally friendly because it uses less land and less water.

- Animal Welfare: By deciding on plant-based options, you help lessen animal suffering and advance moral and humane treatment.

- Food Justice: Adopt a plant-based diet as a means of resolving issues with unfair access to wholesome and sustainable food sources.

- Consider supporting or participating in advocacy efforts that support a plant-based diet, environmental sustainability, and animal welfare.

Keep in mind that your transition to a plant-based diet is unique to you and flexible. To develop a plant-based lifestyle that is sustainable, fulfilling, and in line with your values and health objectives, gradually incorporate these suggestions and techniques.

Chapter 9: Success Stories and Testimonials

In this chapter, we highlight the inspiring tales of people who adopted a plant-based diet in an effort to live a healthier and more environmentally friendly lifestyle. Anyone considering or already embracing the advantages of a plant-based diet can find inspiration and motivation from their individual journeys.

9.1 Authentic Transformations

These are accounts of actual people who adopted a plant-based diet and saw amazing changes in their lives:

John's Weight Loss Experience: For years, John, a software engineer, had trouble with his weight. He made the decision to change his diet and adopt a plant-based one. John lost more than 60 pounds by engaging in regular exercise and eating whole, plant-based foods. His energy levels increased, and he no longer required blood pressure medication.

Sarah's Victory over Health Problems Having three children, Sarah faced a difficult battle with autoimmune diseases that left her feeling worn out and in pain. She changed her diet to a plant-based one, and her symptoms started to get better. She regained her energy and was able to interact with her family in a meaningful way.

9.2 Journeys to a Healthier Lifestyle: Personal Accounts

These life experiences show how adopting a plant-based diet can significantly enhance general health:

Alex's Road to Fitness: To improve his athletic performance, Alex, a gym owner and fitness enthusiast, switched to a plant-based diet. He increased his strength and muscle mass, but he also recovered from workouts more quickly and had less inflammation, which allowed him to push the boundaries of his fitness even further.

Ella's Path to Ethical Eating: Ella, a fervent supporter of animals, decided to adopt a plant-based diet in order to better align her dietary preferences with her moral principles. She started looking into plant-based recipes and eco-friendly products because she is passionate about sustainability and animal welfare.

9.3 Testimonials that Inspire

These touching testimonies demonstrate the profound effects of a plant-based diet on people's lives:

"At first, I was dubious, but my transition to a plant-based diet has been a revelation. I've lost weight without counting calories, my skin has improved, and I feel more energised. Additionally, I now relish cooking delicious plant-based meals for my family. - Lisa

"I've had digestive problems for a long time, and I never felt great after eating. These issues went away when I changed to a plant-based diet. Now that I know I'm nourishing my body and not harming animals, I eat with joy and satisfaction. - David

"I thought it would be impossible to give up cheese and meat, but I couldn't have been more mistaken. There are so many incredible plant-based substitutes, and I've learned about flavors and cuisines I had no idea existed. I feel happier, healthier, and more earth-connected. - Emily

"As a mother, I wanted to give my kids the brightest future possible. I'm teaching my children the value of making sustainable decisions and having compassion for animals by adopting a plant-based diet. - Maria

These success tales and endorsements serve as evidence of how a plant-based diet has the power to alter people's lives. They demonstrate how adopting this way of life can result in significant changes in one's physical, emotional, and moral well-being and encourage all of us to lead healthier, more compassionate lives. The experiences of these people show the beneficial effects a plant-based diet can have on your life and the world around you, regardless of how long you've been on it.

Conclusion

Celebrating Your Plant-Based Journey

As we conclude "The Complete Plant-Based Kitchen Cookbook for Beginners: Nourishing Recipes for a Healthier You," I want to congratulate you on beginning the journey toward a healthier, kinder, and more environmentally conscious way of life. A conscious decision that affects your health, the environment, and even the lives of animals is what your plant-based journey is all about. You've started down a path that will yield many benefits, and I am genuinely optimistic about your future.

You now know how to make delicious, wholesome plant-based meals that are good for your body and your taste buds. You now have a wide variety of recipes to choose from, ranging from colorful salads to filling stews, sweet treats to cool drinks.

Do not forget that this is a marathon, not a sprint. There might be obstacles in your path, but your perseverance, coupled with the information and recipes in this book, will enable you to get past them. Every meal you eat that is made of plants advances your quest for better health.

Further Resources

Consider looking into additional resources to help you on your journey, such as:

Books: There are countless plant-based cookbooks out there, each with its own collection of recipes and information.

Online Communities: Participate in online discussion boards and social media groups to meet like-minded people, exchange stories, and learn about new dishes.

Websites with educational content: Read up on the advantages of a plant-based diet for your health, sustainable living, and moral issues on reputable websites and blogs.

Cooking Classes: To further develop your culinary abilities, think about enrolling in a plant-based cooking class in your neighborhood or online.

Local Farmers' Markets: Shop at your neighborhood farmers' markets to support regional farmers and find fresh, in-season produce.

About the Author

Dr. Adam C. stands as a beacon of inspiration in the fields of medicine, nutrition, and self-help, with a remarkable journey that exemplifies the transformative power of healthy living. Armed with a professional master's degree in health nutrition and years of experience, Dr. C. has become a guiding light for individuals seeking to embrace vibrant well-being and lead happier lives.

From an early age, Dr. C. navigated through a myriad of health challenges that ranged from genetic predispositions to the pitfalls of unhealthy eating. His personal struggle ignited a flame of determination within him, one that was fueled by the belief that the human body possesses an incredible ability to heal and rejuvenate through the right nourishment. Through steadfast dedication, Dr. C. managed to conquer his own ailments and emerged as a living testament to the transformative potential of a well-balanced lifestyle.

What sets Dr. Adam C. apart is his rich tapestry of experiences, having been deeply immersed in groundbreaking research in health food and diet-related domains. His quest to uncover the hidden treasures of nutrients within our meals has led to groundbreaking revel ations that empower individuals to extract the maximum benefit from their dietary choices. Dr. C.'s research has not only contributed to the scientific community but has also served as a roadmap for countless individuals striving to optimize their health.

However, it is not just Dr. C.'s academic prowess that has touched lives it is his unparalleled compassion and empathy that truly make him a beacon of hope. His personal journey of triumph over adversity infuses his guidance with an authentic understanding of the challenges his readers and patients face. Dr. C. doesn't just prescribe nutritional plans; he fosters a deep connection with his audience, instilling in them the confidence to embark on their own transformative journeys.

Dr. Adam C.'s holistic approach reaches beyond the confines of traditional medicine. His insights have translated into self-help resources that empower individuals to take charge of their wellness narrative. His words resonate on paper as they do in person, making his books not mere guides, but trusted companions on the path to vitality.

In the realm of health and nutrition, Dr. C. shines as a true luminary. His core strengths lie in his ability to synthesize complex scientific findings into practical, actionable advice that individuals from all walks of life can seamlessly integrate into their routines. Dr. C.'s legacy is not just a collection of breakthroughs; it is a testament to the extraordinary potential that lies within each of us to overcome obstacles and embrace a life brimming with health, happiness, and fulfillment.

As an experienced doctor, passionate nutritionist, and empathetic author, Dr. Adam C. continues to transform lives, showing us that the journey to a healthier, happier existence is within our grasp, waiting to be unlocked through the power of informed choices and unwavering determination.

www.ingramcontent.com/pod-product-compliance
Lightning Source LLC
Chambersburg PA
CBHW050842260726
48660CB00006B/2392